Talking About Sex: Lean How to Talk With Your Children On Adult Topics

Table of Contents

Introduction

Welcome to Talking To Your Kids about Sex, a book designed to approach your kids about the topic of sex in one of the best ways. A lot of individuals tend to have a hard time talking about sex with their children, but, more importantly, many of them miss talking about some of the most crucial parts about sex. Since this is such a long lasting topic, we'll go over not only how to talk about sex, but also how to prepare your child to properly handle sex with its many risks, dangers, and what they can use to protect themselves. Let's Begin.

Chapter 1 – Making The Conversation Not Awkward

Determining The Correct Time

The problem with having this conversation is that it is extremely uncomfortable from both sides, primarily because parents tend to wait until their kids are in their teenage years in order to have this conversation. They like to cover it up until then and hide it from their kids as much as possible, but most tend to forget that they usually knew about it far before their parents ever thought it was the correct time for the sex talk. Here's a tip for those who don't realize this, if sex is already uncomfortable to talk about then you have already gone past the point where sex is alright to talk about.

The issue is that sex is treated as a taboo subject, which is why it is hidden most households. However, there is a trend when it comes to handling subjects with children that presents itself in the most extreme cases. The longer you go without talking about something, the more potential damage that something can have on a child's life. A child who is sheltered and praised for an enormous portion of their life quickly becomes suicidal when introduced to the outside world while many who are criticized early on find it very easy to transition over. The same can be said about sex in the fact that the longer you go without talking to them about it, the more resistant they will be to the information and advice.

Let Them Watch The Bad Movies... Some of Them

Odds are that you have been following a rating system, either the one that has been put in place or by one that you set. The problem is that human interactions don't have this rating, and, well, life does not have this rating. As much as you may try, you will not be able to prevent them from finding out, which is why it is best for you to be the one that introduces it early on in a controlled situation. While you may not allow them to watch the truly horrible movies, movies that provide soft porn or sex that is not explicitly shown on the television or even just kissing, you should use a medium to begin introducing the topic to them.

This will be uncomfortable for them as not only are they being introduced to something that they view as "gross" at the time, but they are watching the taboo subject with you, the parent. Once you have noticed that they are not glancing at you to make sure they can watch this every five seconds, you can now rest assured they feel comfortable about the topic. The age to ideally start this is around ten to eleven years old or about the time they are in the sixth or seventh grade.

Changing Thinking Patterns

There's a lot to be said about telling a child to not ask questions or telling them they are not ready when it deals with a bad subject. When dealing with big, life-changing topics you need to be open to questions and admit when you don't know something. The more open you are about talking about something, the less their little minds will crave to know everything they can to know about it.

The problem with most parents is the fact that they haven't had to experience what it was like to not know what something was about and be pressured by the consequences of a taboo act. It feels good to go against the grain when you are young and consequences are not very high on the list of concerns because kids are often taught they should be more worried about the punishment of their parents over the punishment of their own actions. What do I mean by this? Why is a child most likely not going to voluntarily touch a hot stove but more than willing to steal something of immediate value if they know they'll likely get away with it?

The first consequence is if the child touches a hot stove, they see themselves as causing themselves pain. The second consequence is a challenge in that if they can get away with it then this is their reward. Therefore, the second is more akin to a game since it is a challenge and we all know how addicting games can be. This leads us to the next chapter.

Chapter 2 – Introducing the Conversation

Don't Talk, Do Show

There's a lot to be said about allowing a child to live through a simulation of their end result. This was the primary thinking of having a child taking care of a baby of something for an extended period of time. The problem with this type of thinking is that it does not take several factors into the equation:

- A child doesn't have to worry about whether it will starve or not when it lives with parents.

- Usually, the program was gender-biased.

- Usually, the program only had one gender taking care of the child.

- Usually, the program never mentioned anything about bills.

The list goes on and on about the differences between a real-life situation versus a simulation of it. Taking care of a fake child when you have all the materials at the ready is not difficult. What happens if they refuse to do it? They get reprimanded and nothing actually happens. That's a huge problem because if a parent actually refuses to take care of a child, they have to face a lot more than a slap on the wrist. Such a program backfired and seemingly caused more pregnancies because it usually gave the kids false confidence.

A True Program

You don't even need to give them a fake baby to do this. All you need to do is give them "a paycheck" and start billing them. You start them out by calculating the actual amount they cost you to live there, including food, internet, and what not. The more work they do around the house, the more their imaginary dollars go up.

The less work they do, the more their imaginary dollars go down. Introducing them to this model, you can then start having them handle their own bills for a little while before introducing a baby into the mix. The actual rewards of what they can get for their "more dollars" is up to you, but taking away their entertainment (like credit card companies do when you can't pay their bills) is a good way to motivate them to earn "more dollars". The idea of this type of program, is to get them to build up a savings to take care of their own child. It is also very important to let them know that this is the intention of the program, otherwise they will believe they have to do this until they are old enough to move out.

Once you introduce a baby into the mix, take them to the actual products they would buy in a store and have them calculate how much they need to make extra. You really only should do this for the first month or until they have no more in their savings. The amount of money it takes to take care of a child should quickly overwhelm them, which is the point of such a program. It should bring them to the realization that children cost a lot of money and that the fate of children are tied to their parents. If you want the impact to be huge and shocking, you could include the price of giving birth. I know a child costs around $25,000 just to be born these days.

Starting The Talk

If you chose not to follow any of the previous advice, then you can go ahead with this step anyway. The conversation has to come up naturally, as in it cannot be introduced out of nowhere because this is what makes the conversation awkward. Going back to some advice given in the first chapter, letting them watch a somewhat inappropriate movie and pausing the inappropriate scene is usually a good way to start this conversation.

The issue with going ahead with an awkward conversation is that the child will be more resistant to the information that you give. Our brains are relational, which means the best way they retain something is when they can immediately relate the information it is being given to something that is already stored in their mind. If a brain is introduced to a topic without any reason as to why it is occurring in that moment, the brain will only accept information that it can use to get out of that moment. By providing visual material to tie it to, you can open the brain up to receive and embed more of the knowledge for future use.

Do Not Try To Relate

If you have ever looked at the common lingo between your child and their friends and wondered what a good portion of it meant, you are not the only parent to do so. You immediately understand that you cannot relate to that speech, so why is it that you are compelled to relate to your child's sex life? The issue is that your brain is trying to come from a relational standpoint, as that is the best way we can explain difficult topics but this is not the best way to teach. We don't teach children by telling them what their parents would do, we show examples of what works and doesn't work. Therefore, the best way to talk about sex to a child is give tell them what you have done; what worked and what didn't work.

There are a few reasons why you should do this. First, it comes in as a storytelling aspect and makes the child want to ask more questions about why you did certain things. Secondly, because you are telling stories, the atmosphere of the conversation changes completely from awkward to interest. Thirdly, it will show your child what succeeds and what fails in a situation where sex is involved. Mind you, this is only to start the conversation and you should open up plenty of time for this conversation because it will be a long one.

Chapter 3 – Health Talk

While it is important to help a child understand sex and the end result of normal sex, you will need to eventually get to the point of talking to them about health. Since STD's are only transmitted by sex and some STD's have telling signs, you should cover this area when the questioning begins. However, there are some key things you should do when you have this conversation.

Don't Act Like You Know Everything

The problem most parents and a good portion of educators is that they tend to act like they know everything. In this education's day and age, the teach seems to have all the answers in front of the students. Meanwhile, they have to Google what the kids are talking about some of the time on their computers to make sure they know what it means. This is a bad habit because it forces kids into a corner where they are less resourceful on their own and you see this result in a lot of children who find their first job but almost always stay at it longer than they should.

The problem with sex in acting like you know everything is that you not only set your child up to miss something important, but you set yourself up for a similar fumble. The internet is the greatest resource for knowledge of all time, which means that if your child has a question you can't answer then you both should be Google'ing it. You should also give a valid reason as to why you trust the websites you land on for the answer to the question (which should not be "It was the first one there"). Setting this example engrains into your child that when you don't know something, you should *research* the answer. This has been taught **out** of kids so much that when they have to go to higher levels of learning, they have to relearn how to learn on their own. Their teachers and parents have always either told them to be quiet or had the answer for them, so most children don't know how to learn on their own properly. Additionally, telling the child why you trust specific websites tells them that not all websites or information on the internet holds true because a lot of children believe this until it is entirely too late.

More Gross Equals Better Education

This is often glossed over, but if you plan on talking about sex with your child then you should go for the grossest things possible in every corner. This is a technique that is mastered by the devoutly religious, as you see they and their children tend to follow the teachings to the teeth. If you show them the most horrible thing that can happen to themselves as a result of their actions, they are far more likely to give it a second thought when the opportunity arises.

The reason why this is effective is the body works in the favor of what will make more survival sense rather than what would make more common sense. The point of the reproduction system makes sure that the child will attempt to have intercourse at one time or more, but the brain includes risks in its equation. Therefore, if you show the risks of contracting a disease specifically given through sex, it provides the brain with more reason why it should be hesitant in doing so. If it is backed by authorities, or people that your child see as authorities, the value of that risk increases exponentially. That is because children are often shown that authorities are individuals that are worth trusting in order to ensure the continued survival of self, the primary goal of the human body. Thus, the more risk you show to the mind, the more likely your child will be careful about who they choose to have sex with.

Talk About Situational Awareness

Perhaps the longest running buttend of a joke about sex is based on having sex in the back of a car, which is something I've never understood. I mean, how short do you have to be in order for that to actually work? The average car doesn't even let you fully lay out in the back for some rest, let alone provide a large enough area for sex. It's just a thing people say to say or a thing people who have trucks/ obscenely big vehicles.

This brings up the next point; making sure they understand the importance of paying attention to their surroundings when they have uncontrollable urges. The number one mental picture that pops up about sex is a bedroom, but, in reality, there are far more places to have sex than the car or the bedroom. Movies show this all the time, like the seats underneath a stadium or the maintenance closet in nearly every hospital show.

The truth about this, from a medical perspective, is horrifying. That's like going pee in the community pool. You don't think much about it until you realize there might be some fluid exchange happening you don't know about. Paying attention in where you have sex can prevent a lot of unforeseen consequences. Pointing out a child that someone with A.I.D.s could have been the last person to have sex in an area of a public place is a quick way to get them to think twice about where they have sex. After all, if they found it then what's to say someone else didn't find it before them. While this may seem ridiculous, a number of cases show support that having sex in an area where a diseased person previously stayed can transmit that disease the person had.

Chapter 4 – Hidden Consequences

This chapter will be divided into two different sections: male and female. This is due to the fact that the genders are affected by hormones differently and, therefore, need different advice about what should be done.

Male Advice About Hidden Consequences

Do Not Force A Grandchild

This is, perhaps, one of the most damaging things you could do for a child's sex life. Telling them you just want a grandchild automatically puts stress on them until the time they have a child. Even more so, it adds duplicative stress if you die before that child has a child of their own.

Beyond the added stress, you don't want to force them into this as they may try to do it before they have the money to do it. As we know, having a child is expensive and if they have a child before they're ready to afford it, you can bet that you are likely going to be supporting them. If you don't support them, either they will become a statistic in Child Services or the next decade or more of their life is going to be difficult.

Be Careful of the Women You Hang Out With Alone

As a parent, this may come as a shocker to you but for the men and women who are still sexually active this isn't at all surprising. You have a grand array of psychotic situations to choose from here that are actually common:

- A woman steals seamen off a toilet from a man to impregnate herself and then claims child support.

- A man agrees to stay with a woman, who is not his wife, giving birth to a child, who is not his child, and then ends up paying child support for the child.

- A man is raped by a woman while he is asleep and forced to pay child support when she has a child.

- A man's name is used in place of another man as the father on a certificate. This man is forced, five to ten years after a paternity test proves no genetic relationship, to continue child support payments.

These are actually common and there are no tools in place to stop it any time soon. This is not the end of the list of difficult situations actively sexual men have to deal with on a regular basis and almost no parent prepares their children to face these types of women.

There is Little to No Current Help For Single Fathers

There is no M.I.C. where there is a W.I.C. to help support a child. When you request Food Stamps as a father, the mother's name is usually the main account holder. If divorced or separated, a father can lose the children if he tries to collect help from the government whereas a mother just has to say the father isn't paying child support and the government goes after the father for money. This is not to be confused in saying that a father can't do the same, it is just that fathers tend to lose rights to their children after they have made the request. You will find hundreds, if not thousands, of single mother scholarships but it's doubtful you could collect even ten single father scholarships. There are virtually no help shelters for abused men in relationships while there are thousands for women.

Be Mindful In Dress

Don't come at me with that. For women, sexual attraction is almost always in the mind. For men, sexual attraction is almost always visual. You can tell men "not to rape" but it only does so good. There are men who ignore these laws and we call them criminals because words didn't stop them. That doesn't mean you should tell them to be a Puritan, but they should be aware that certain areas of a city require a certain type of dress code to stay relatively safe in. It's not the woman's fault, it never is, but dressing a certain way can make her stand out among other women who might have also become a victim in that circumstance. It's not an ideal reality, but it is what it is.

Learn How To Fight

Most victims only learn how to fight after an incident has happened, which makes it close to pointless. Learning how to defend yourself, as boys mostly do naturally among themselves, is vitally important for ensuring that sex is never forced on them. It's also very important the type of fighting they're taught as they should learn something like Aikido or Brazilian Jujitsu. These are grappling methods of fighting, which makes them very useful for those who are weak and for those who are currently pinned to the ground.

Be Careful of Male Friends

Most rape occurs with males who are relatively close to a woman, such as a brother or a male friend. These men usually obsess about the woman to the point where they can no longer control their urges and attack the woman. It's not all men, but they should still be careful about staying alone with men who are overly fond of them as this is normally the first sign of an attraction. Gathering a group of friends that are more female than male is a great way to prevent this as rapists are usually lone gunners and won't attack when there's more people in the group than just you and them. More so, having more females than males also prevents group raping, which is common in scenarios where the men are overly confident and abrasive.

Chapter 5 – Protection

At some point, amidst all the lovely graphical images planted in their head, they will ask about how to protect themselves if they don't already know. This is where there are multiple options for both males and females, but you have to just list them for your child and this is another area where parents sometimes slip up on the information the child actually needs by telling them what worked for them rather than just letting them know what all is out there.

Contraceptives (With men too, don't just skip past this one)

That's right, for a long time women have had access to contraceptives but more recently, as in the past five years of releasing this book, men also have access to contraceptives and it's an exploding market right now. Sure, the first option for nearly everyone is a condom but condoms break, people are allergic to them now, and sometimes it's just cheaper to go with the pill for the few of us who are Spartacus or Wonder Woman in bed.

However, that's not the only thing you need to tell them as they will likely just hear "the pill that lets me have all the unprotected sex" part and not listen to anything else. The pill comes with a few side effects. After all, it's affecting one of the core functions in our bodies that runs off of hormones and blood. Problems such as heart failure, a break out in rashes, and becoming permanently impotent are vital issues to talk about.

The Almighty Condom

It's been around since 1844. Yes, the condom has been around for over a hundred years and it is still the most common way to protect oneself from impregnation of the female gender. However, it comes with some drawbacks, the first of which is the feeling and this is the most difficult part. Men like to go raw because it feels better, but, at the same time, they run a serious risk of impregnating a woman. There are still no laws that protect a man when the woman decides she doesn't want an abortion and it's a social stigma to even suggest that a man having a similar choice to a woman in terms of reproductivity is equality. Therefore, without a man's version of an abortion, men are left with the tools left to them for over a hundred years.

The second drawback is that some women are allergic to every condom, or even most of them, which makes it nearly impossible to have any choice of protection in sex. The final drawback is that companies can go cheap on the product, which leads to some VERY RARE incidents where the condom breaks and we all know how that story ends. However, what is important to convey to the children is the fact that condoms not only help protect against impregnation, but also help against certain types of STD's and that's why people shouldn't solely rely on contraceptives.

Conclusion

Welcome to the end of this book. We've gone over a lot of material and a lot of controversial material at that. We've gone over some of the unfair things that women and men have to face whenever they engage in sex along with how to get your children used to being more open about the topic with you.

As always, this book is not meant to complete all of your knowledge on this topic, but rather boost what you may already know or give you a good footing on the topic before you tackle it. We may be done with this book, but, for now, good luck.

FREE Bonus Reminder

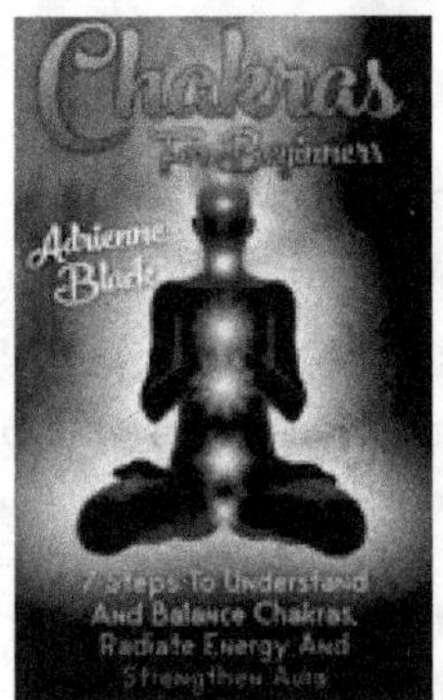

If you have not grabbed it yet, please go ahead and download your special bonus E book *"Chakras for Beginners. 7 Steps To Understand And Balance Chakras, Radiate Energy, And Strengthen Aura"*.

Simply Click the Button Below

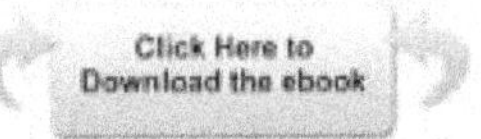

OR **Go to This Page**

http://lifehacksworld.com/free

BONUS #2: More Free & Discounted Books & Products

Do you want to receive more Free/Discounted Books or Products?

We have a mailing list where we send out our new Books or Products when they go free or with a discount on Amazon. Click on the link below to sign up for Free & Discount Book & Product Promotions.

=> Sign Up for Free & Discount Book & Product Promotions <=

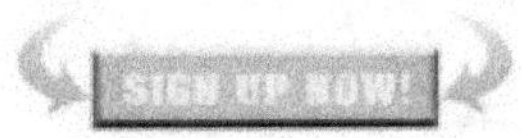

OR Go to this URL

http://zbit.ly/1WBb1Ek

9 781721 117673